A DRINKING PROBLEM

may well find its source in an eating problem. Studies of alcoholics have shown that they have unique nutritional needs, and that their condition is often brought about by special nutritional deficiencies and/or allergies. Changes in diet and specifically tailored nutritional supplementation — notably with vitamin B3, though other nutrients play vital roles — have brought about up to 80 percent recovery rates for even long-term alcoholics and problem drinkers — far greater than those accomplished by conventional therapies.

This guide to the nutritional nature and treatment of alcoholism and problem drinking contains the latest research and a basic program of diet and vitamin/mineral supplementation.

ABOUT THE AUTHOR AND EDITORS

Ruth M. Guenther, Ph.D., has a special interest in the relationship between nutrition and behavior, ever since her discovery of her own connection with junk food and hypoglycemia. A one-and-a-half year study with alcoholics at a veteran's medical center in Texas resulted in her dissertation for her doctorate: *The Effect of Nutritional Therapy on Rehabilitation of Alcoholics.* She is a statistician with the Texas Adult Probation Commission, and has published articles in the *Texas Journal of Correction* and *Perspectives* on nutrition and alcoholism which might well influence the future treatment of that widespread disease.

Richard A. Passwater, Ph.D., is one of the most called-upon authorities for information relating to preventive health care. A noted biochemist, he is credited with popularizing the term "supernutrition" largely as a result of having written two bestsellers on the subject—*Supernutrition: Megavitamin Revolution* and *Supernutrition for Healthy Hearts.* His other books include *Easy No-Flab Diet, Cancer and Its Nutritional Therapies,* and the recently published *Selenium as Food & Medicine.* He has just completed a new book on hair analysis with Elmer M. Cranton, M.D.

Earl Mindell, R.Ph., Ph.D., combines the expertise and working experience of a pharmacist with extensive knowledge in most of the nutrition areas. His book *Earl Mindell's Vitamin Bible* is now a million-copy bestseller; and his more recent *Vitamin Bible for Your Kids* may very well duplicate his first *Bible's* publishing history. Dr. Mindell's popular *Quick & Easy Guide to Better Health* was just published by Keats Publishing.

A NUTRITIONAL GUIDE FOR THE PROBLEM DRINKER

THE LATEST RESEARCH ON THE EFFECT OF PROPER DIET AND VITAMIN/MINERAL SUPPLEMENTATION IN REMEDYING ALCOHOL ABUSE

by Ruth M. Guenther, Ph.D.

Keats Publishing, Inc. New Canaan, Connecticut

A Nutritional Guide for the Problem Drinker is not intended as medical advice. Its intention is solely informational and educational. Please consult a medical or health professional should the need for one be warranted. It is important to emphasize this in a booklet on alcoholism since a reaction to withdrawal from alcohol can be so severe as to cause death in some cases.

A NUTRITIONAL GUIDE FOR THE PROBLEM DRINKER

ISBN: 0-87983-295-9

Printed in the United States of America

Good Health Guides are published by Keats Publishing, Inc.
27 Pine Street (Box 876)
New Canaan, Connecticut 06840

Contents

A NUTRITIONAL GUIDE FOR THE PROBLEM DRINKER

THE HIGH COST OF ALCOHOLISM

Alcoholism and alcohol abuse impose a staggering drain on this country, both in lives and economic losses. The full extent of the alcoholism problem is not known, but the following are some widely quoted statistics:

- About 7 percent of our adult population or about 9 million adults are alcoholics.
- Ten percent of the work force are alcoholics representing a 19.6 billion dollar annual loss in productivity.[1,2]
- Alcohol is implicated in 75 - 80 percent of all crime.[3]
- Alcoholism is a major factor in highway deaths.
- Alcoholism is the fourth most common disease seen by physicians.
- Cirrhosis of the liver ranks seventh among leading causes of death.[4]
- Alcohol use and abuse is a growing problem among school age children.

These factors are sufficient in themselves to make alcoholism an important current problem. Of even greater importance is the impact that alcoholism is having on future generations. Consumption of three or more ounces of alcohol per day by a pregnant woman may cause full fetal alcohol syndrome. Consumption of much smaller amounts may cause an increase in the abnormalities classified as minimum brain dysfunction, manifested in children with learning disabilities.[5]

All factors considered, the net effects of alcohol consumption may be even greater than generally suspected. The alcoholism problem deserves not only serious attention but a new approach to prevention and treatment.

THE FAILURE OF CONVENTIONAL CONCEPTS REGARDING ALCOHOLISM

Within the conventional framework, many theories for the cause or causes of alcoholism have arisen. These theories have been in the domain of either psychology or sociology. A survey of the literature on conventional approaches to alcoholism shows that research has failed to find sufficient quantitative evidence to support these theories. Moreover, none of these conventional theories seem to be able to explain why one person becomes an alcoholic while another under similar circumstances does not become an alcoholic.

Many conventional treatment methods for alcoholism have been developed in conjunction with the conventional theories as to the cause or causes of this disease. Conventional treatment methods can be grouped into the following general categories: psychological treatment, institutional treatment, social or group therapy such as Alcoholics Anonymous, and chemotherapy such as tranquilizers or antabuse. In actual practice, most conventional treatment methods consist of some combination of these types.

However, differences in treatment methodology do not appear to significantly affect recovery from alcoholism.[6,7] Prognosis for alcoholics undergoing conventional alcoholism treatment is poor. Recidivism rates (the percentage of alcoholics resuming drinking following discharge from treatment) appear to range from 65 to 75 percent. That is, two-thirds to three-fourths of all alcoholics undergoing conventional treatment can be expected to return to drinking within a relatively short time. The outlook is probably worse on a long-term basis, and the recidivism rate may be much higher — possibly 95 percent — if a longer period after discharge were taken into account.

THE DISEASE CONCEPT OF ALCOHOLISM

A fundamental reason for the failure of conventional treatment methods may lie in the failure of most alcoholic rehabilitation professionals to treat alcoholism as if it were the disease it really is. In spite of the millions of dollars that have been spent on alcoholism research, alcoholism has never been clearly defined nor have the criteria for distinguishing who is an alcoholic been firmly established. The only agreement seems to be the central assumption of loss of control, with accompanying involuntary and excessive drinking.

Nevertheless, alcoholism truly is a disease — one which results in acquired and increased tissue tolerance, inability to abstain from drinking, and withdrawal symptoms so severe as to cause death in some cases. Further, excessive drinking causes a disorder that may be called addiction, implying a pharmacological disorder. Alcohol has the capacity to produce physical and mental abnormalities consistent with the concept of disease and involving sufficient numbers of people to be considered an epidemic by some authorities.

It is a commonly accepted notion that diseases are treated by members of the medical profession. Is it not curious, then, that alcoholism is the only disease for which a patient is commonly referred by physicians to a lay organization — that is, to Alcoholics Anonymous — for treatment? Other alcoholics may find themselves referred to alcoholic rehabilitation units headed by psychologists and staffed by counselors (often themselves recovering alcoholics) and one or more social workers. Neither psychologists nor social workers qualify as healers of disease. Finally, much of the research into the cause or causes of alcoholism has been conducted by psychologists or sociologists rather than by biochemists or medical researchers.

The failure of most practitioners in alcoholism treatment to recognize alcoholism primarily as a disease of the body and only secondarily as a problem in social or psychological maladjustment is basic to the failure of conventional treatment methods.

BIOCHEMISTRY AND ALCOHOLISM

During the past three decades, studies have been performed which link alcoholism to biochemistry in various ways. Allergies, excessive use of caffeine, hypoglycemia, and heredity have all been implicated as possible biochemical factors.

Alcoholism as an allergic response. Allergy and addiction, long considered as separate phenomena, have been hypothesized recently to be different manifestations of the same disorder. The difference occurs in the timing of the symptoms. An allergic response is usually immediate. On the other hand, the reaction could be delayed (masked) by eating the food to which the person is allergic, thereby temporarily relieving the symptoms. The term "addiction" has been applied to this masked food allergy. The addiction reaction appears as a withdrawal symptom, occurring at varying time intervals ranging from several hours to days, depending on the severity of the addiction/allergy. Thus alcoholism may be an addiction to a favorite alcoholic beverage caused by allergy to the food from which the alcohol is made.[8] Other researchers have speculated that alcoholism may be an allergic response to the congeners in the alcohol (those impurities from the aging process carried over in the distillation process). The allergic reaction is said to cause the hangover symptoms.[9]

Allergic reactions may result from biochemical defects, either inherited or acquired. If the latter, they may be the body's reaction to stress. The more deranged the biochemistry, the more numerous will be the allergic responses exhibited. As good health is restored through sound nutritional practices, allergic reactions should gradually diminish and eventually disappear.[10]

Alcoholism and caffeine consumption. Caffeine and alcohol are probably the most widely used psychotropic drugs in North America. An intriguing relationship between caffeine and alcohol consumption was postulated in which high daily caffeine consumption and dietary imbalance may lead to heavy alcohol consumption in the evening.[11] Investigation of the effect of caffeine on voluntary alcohol consumption by rats indicated that alcohol consumption increased slowly but substantially when caffeine was added to a diet that was only marginally inadequate; that is, one that provided sufficient calories while being deficient in protein, vitamins and minerals, not unlike the typical American diet. Alcohol consumption fell to pre-caffeine levels as soon as caffeine was withdrawn.[12] Support for this relationship is found in studies which have noted the high consumption of coffee by alcoholics.

Alcoholism and hypoglycemia. Increasing evidence is beginning to show that faulty sugar metabolism which causes a condition known as hypoglycemia (low blood sugar) may be implicated in alcoholism. Whether or not hypoglycemia is involved in a causal mechanism, it is known that hypoglycemia can result from heavy alcohol consumption. The craving of recovering alcoholics for sugary foods is well known.

Alcoholism and heredity. In support of a genetic component, Dr. Roger Williams has suggested a genetotrophic disease principle as a precipitating factor in alcoholism.[13] A "genetotrophic condition" in medicine refers to a condition predisposed by heredity and precipitated by nutritional factors. Williams's genetotrophic theory states that basic nutritional needs are determined by an inherited metabolic machinery. Phenylketonuria is an example of a genetotrophic disease in which an inherited defective enzyme pattern does not permit proper metabolism of tryptophan. Stringent control of an infant's diet can prevent severe mental retardation.

According to Dr. Williams, the fundamental condition relating alcoholism to biochemistry and nutrition is a unique, innate, and highly distinctive biochemical individuality.[14] Dr. Williams's repeated stress on the factor of biochemical individuality is crucial to the understanding of his genetotrophic theory. Research has shown that monozygous animals with similar gene pools have major anatomical and biochemical differences. If animals having similar gene pools show wide variation, the notion of even more distinctive constitutional patterns in humans who have widely diverse genetic patterns becomes compelling.[15]

Because of this disparity in human biochemistry, nutritional needs among individuals may vary as much as a hundred to a thousand times. Thus the notion that nutrition is concerned only in "deficiency" diseases such as pellagra, in which the deficiency is overt — that is, clinically diagnosable — is no longer defensible. It is also incorrect to assume that alcoholics become malnourished only as a result of their alcoholism. There is a growing body of evidence to show that nutritional requirements of alcoholics are quite different from those of non-alcoholics.[16] The crucial factor relating alcoholism to biochemistry and nutrition is that alcoholics have unmet nutritional needs prior to becoming alcoholics, predisposing them to alcoholism. For these persons, nutrition is of the utmost importance. Williams stated: "Diet quality has far reaching influence including effect on food choice and reactions to surgery and poisons. One may wonder what is not related to nutrition." Williams was referring to supernutrition — total nutrition in its most sophisticated sense in which quality of diet rather than simply sufficient calories is the overriding concern.[17]

Animal studies have indicated that voluntary alcohol consumption can be turned on and off repeatedly by changes in nutrition. In addition to vitamin deficiencies, changes in sugar and fat content of an animal's diet were shown to cause changes in alcohol consumption.[18]

In another study, animals kept on a vitamin-rich diet during the first two-thirds of their lives did not consume as much alcohol when placed on an inadequate diet as rats kept on a vitamin-poor diet during the first two-thirds of their lives and then offered alcohol. Thus childhood nutrition may be a precipitating factor in alcoholism.[19]

Constitutional or psychological stress can substantially alter body chemistry and impair cellular functioning. Particularly involved are those cells having to do with regulating appetites, probably located in the hypothalamus region of the brain. Since stress is known to drastically increase the need for certain nutrients, stress may well be a precipitating factor in alcoholism. However, the body's wisdom in regulating appetite or food choices can no longer be relied upon.[10,14]

Vulnerability to alcohol may begin with stress, which may create a desire for alcohol. With each succeeding drink, a person's nutritional needs increase tremendously. The reason for this great increase in nutritional need is that alcohol not only replaces wholesome food but of itself supplies only naked calories. That is, although alcohol becomes a source of energy, it is totally devoid of nutrients. Metabolizing the alcohol further reduces the body's nutritional stores. The body is left with a net deficit in nutrients that grows increasingly larger with each succeeding drink. Furthermore, research has shown that the ability of a drinker's body to absorb nutrients is greatly diminished.[20] Therefore, because of an alcoholic's innate larger-than-average nutritional requirements and acquired nutritional deficiencies, diet is particularly important. In choosing food, however, the emphasis must always be on the quality of food and not simply calories.

Further support of genetic factors in predisposition to alcoholism has been shown in twin studies and studies of familial alcoholism. Results of twin studies indicate a significant genetic factor contributing not only to frequency and regularity of drinking but also to the amount of alcohol consumed. A high prevalance of alcoholism is frequently noted among relatives of alcoholics. In addition, where there was alcoholism in the family, recovering alcoholics tended to resume drinking at a higher rate than alcoholics with a history of little or no familial alcoholism.[21]

Williams's theory, suggesting both cause and treatment, comes closest to conceptualizing alcoholism as a disease by suggesting pre-alcoholic constitutional factors which may lead to a larger than average intake of alcohol. In contrast to the conventional theories discussed earlier, Dr. Williams's genetotrophic theory explains why one person can become an alcoholic while another person in a similar circumstance may not. It is not the circumstance which causes the alcoholism but the uniqueness of the individual's inherited biochemistry and the individual's biochemical response to that circumstance that is crucial to the alcoholism.

From Dr. Williams's and other biochemical theories has grown the concept of nutritional therapy. Nutritional therapy seeks to restore the biochemical balance in the body by nutritional means, including the use of vitamin and mineral supplements according to individual need. The fact that there is no barrier between the body and the brain is frequently overlooked in conventional alcoholism treatment. Biochemical theories make clear, on the other hand, that behavior cannot be considered as a separate entity from the physical body. Implicit within this framework is that restoration of the biochemical balance in the body will normalize behavior.

NUTRITIONAL THERAPY

Nutritional therapy for treatment of alcoholism was an outgrowth of the successful use of vitamin B3 for treatment of schizophrenia. In 1952, Drs. Hoffer and Osmond first introduced the use of massive doses of niacin (vitamin B3) as a treatment for schizophrenia. This treatment proved astonishingly successful. A few interested physicians joined Hoffer and Osmond in using B3 therapy for rehabilitation. Throughout the years that followed, a growing number of not only schizophrenics but also alcoholic schizophrenics were successfully rehabilitated. Treatment was usually limited to massive doses of B3 alone or B3 was given along with a limited number of other vitamins and minerals. The dosage varied but the amount administered was considerably larger than that considered necessary by conventional medical authorities for life and health. Also part of the treatment was a hypoglycemia-controlling diet; that is, a high-protein, low-carbohydrate diet with no caffeine, alcohol, or refined sugar allowed.[22]

Reports have been published indicating that wherever this treatment method has been used, the results have been strikingly more effective than conventional methods in rehabilitating alcoholics. Recovery rates of 75 to 80 percent have been reported, in stark contrast to the 75 percent recidivism rates reported for conventional alcoholism treatment.

However, this concept of orthomolecular or nutritional

therapy as applied to alcoholics offers a very limited view of the nutritional requirements of most alcoholics for several reasons. First, most alcoholics do not eat well when they are drinking heavily. Therefore they require a much more broadly based vitamin and mineral supplementation than that offered by the treatment described above.[14] Second, use of a high protein, low-carbohydrate diet without regard to the source of the protein may not be sound treatment for alcoholics suffering from possible liver damage. Too much protein, particularly from animal sources, may be difficult for the liver to detoxify, especially a liver already damaged from alcohol abuse.[16] Third, research has shown that persons who have difficulty metabolizing refined carbohydrates such as sugar and white flour can readily manage wholegrain products. If non-processed food is used, limiting the amount of carbohydrate in the diet may be unnecessary.[23] There is an added advantage to using whole grains, since these foods also provide excellent sources of more desirable, non-animal protein.

The elimination of sugar, caffeine, cigarettes, and obviously alcohol from the diet should be carefully adhered to. Research with alcoholics indicated unusual sensitivity to caffeine and sugar. Withdrawal of these two substances brought feelings of relaxation and calmness.[21] Smoking has not only been linked to lung cancer and decreased life span, it is also known to use up large quantities of vitamin C.

A nutritional guide for problem drinkers. Nutrition is a subject about which there is high interest and little agreement. Daily newspapers and popular magazines print frequent but contradictory articles on such topics as the "basic four" food groups, choice of processed or unprocessed foods, and level of vitamin and mineral supplements that may be required. It is true that cellular metabolism is not yet completely understood and, because of wide-ranging individual needs, no hard and fast rules can be stated concerning any one person's requirements or the nutritional requirements of any special group. Nevertheless, each of us can become knowledgeable enough about nutrition to keep ourselves and our families mentally and physically healthy.

Food choices are intensely personal involving deeply entrenched eating habits and tastes. But dietary patterns can be changed while still acknowledging individual and family food preferences. It is essential that the entire family participate in this process.

The remainder of this booklet will introduce some thoughts on dietary patterns for good nutrition. Also included is a *Recommended Reading List.* These books, all paperbacks and readily available, contain much more information on the topics discussed here.

BASIC CONCEPTS OF GOOD NUTRITION

Food can no longer be thought of as providing only energy necessary for metabolism. Food must also supply nutrients for growth, repair, and maintenance of body tissues.

What are nutrients? Nutrients are the building blocks of the human body necessary for growth, maintenance, and repair of body tissue, for regulating body processes, and for energy.[24]

Nutrients belong to groups of proteins, fats, carbohydrates, vitamins and minerals. Water and fiber, although non-nutritive, are also necessary to life. More than forty essential nutrients have been identified. All must be present in appropriate quantities and at the appropriate time to build a sound structure.[10,14,25]

PROTEINS. Many different proteins are required to perform vital body processes. These proteins are made up of twenty-two amino acids which the body assembles in varying proportions. The human body can synthesize fourteen of these amino acids from fragments of food. However, our bodies cannot synthesize the other eight, called essential amino acids. If any one of the eight is missing, protein synthesis will be greatly diminished, perhaps halted. Not only must all eight be present, they must be present in the right proportions. For example, if one of the essential amino acids is present in only half of the amount needed while the remaining seven are present in the full amount needed, the body will utilize only one-half of the seven essential amino acids and discard the rest.[25]

Since amino acid reserves are depleted within a few hours, the body's supply of protein must be renewed several times daily. A sound nutritional program should provide each of these essential amino acids at every meal in the right proportions needed for protein synthesis.[25]

Amino acid patterns of food proteins vary considerably. The "biological value" of a food is given according to how closely a food protein resembles that which the body can use. Essential amino acid patterns of animal protein, egg, and milk protein more nearly match the protein requirements of the human body than do essential amino acid patterns of plant foods. Nevertheless, if a variety of plant proteins are chosen which have complementary amino acid patterns; and if milk, cheese, and eggs are used, the amino acid content of one food can fill in the amino acid deficiency of another food and a meal can be obtained that has a higher biological value than one containing only meat protein.[25]

Americans are brought up to think that one can never get too much protein. The average recommended daily amount is approximately 70 grams (varying somewhat depending on one's body weight). If high quality protein is eaten, approximately 45 grams is all that may be necessary. However, the amount of protein needed will vary not only according to protein quality but also according to individual differences. Since alcohol impairs the body's ability to absorb nutrients, 45 grams can only be regarded as a general guideline. Health of skin, hair and nails, and the speed with which cuts and abrasions heal are all good indicators of protein sufficiency. Observing your body's response to changes in nutrition is extremely important.[25]

VITAMINS AND MINERALS. Vitamins and minerals are also important for proper cellular functioning. At least six major minerals, ten trace minerals, and fourteen vitamins are known to be essential to health. Meats are not necessarily as good providers of vitamins and minerals as plant foods and dairy sources. Most plant foods, if fresh and unprocessed, supply enough nutrients for growth, repair and maintenance of body tissues. As amino acid patterns of proteins vary, plant foods also vary in their vitamin and mineral content. The most complete supply of vitamins and minerals can be obtained only by eating fresh, unprocessed plant foods; that is, vegetables, legumes, and grains.[14]

FATS. Fats are broken down during digestion to form fatty acids. Even if no fats are eaten, the body can synthesize some fatty acids from other foods. However, there are three fatty acids that the body cannot make, called essential fatty acids. Vegetable oils are the principal sources of essential fatty acids with evening primrose oil and safflower oil containing the highest amounts. Recent research has shown that processing vegetable oils causes structural changes of essential fatty acids, affecting utilization. Only vegetable oils that have been refined as little as possible should be used.[26]

CARBOHYDRATES. Carbohydrates are the starches and sugars that constitute the bulk of our diet. Ordinarily thought of as providing only calories or energy, this simplistic approach is dangerous because it promotes the use of white sugar and white flour. The best sources of carbohydrates are fresh, unprocessed plant foods. These foods are broken down slowly in the digestive process, producing a slow, steady stream of energy and nutrients to the body. Your size, activity level, and how well you absorb food will regulate the amount of calories you need.

FIBER. In recent years, the importance of fiber to health has been increasingly recognized. Fiber is not only necessary to move the food along the digestive tract. Fiber has also been reported to increase absorption of nutrients, an important factor for alcoholics whose absorption has been impaired. In addition to whole, unprocessed foods, bran can be added to the diet to provide additional fiber.

Food processing and nutrient loss. Dr. Henry Schroeder has documented the many nutritional inadequacies of the American diet. His studies led him to conclude that although raw foods supply adequate amounts of nutrients, the "typical" American diet, consisting in large part of refined, canned and otherwise processed foods, is marginal.[27]

When food is processed or refined, many nutrients are lost. For example, wholewheat flour is an excellent food. However, during the refining of flour, seven vitamins are depleted to the extent of 50 to 86 percent and thirteen minerals to the extent of 40 to 88 percent. In addition, most of the fiber is lost. The resulting bleached and refined white flour is a very poor source of protein and a very poor source of vitamins and minerals.

Frozen food processors blanch green vegetables with sequestering agents so that a bright green color is obtained later on, when the vegetables are cooked. During blanching, the zinc and manganese content of these vegetables is reduced by 80 percent.[28]

Instant mashed potatoes and canned vegetables also have lost nutrients in processing. Many of the nutrients in canned foods are found in the canning liquid. Unless the liquid is used, most of the food value is discarded when the liquid is thrown away.

Since much nutritive value is lost in processing, it is noteworthy that there are, in most instances, large increases in sodium and sugar. Canned green beans, for example, contain sixty times more salt than the raw food. One brand of cereal contains 3.35 percent by weight of table salt, roughly the salt content of sea water! This same cereal, whose brand name implies that it is 100 percent bran, contains 20 percent by weight of sugar.[29,30]

A prevailing argument in defense of processed food is that whole, fresh, unprocessed foods cost more than processed foods, and consequently the average American cannot afford them. However, if the protein content, the loss of nutritive value due to processing, and the undesirability of large quantities of sugar and salt are taken into consideration, the choice of processed food cannot be justified on the basis of either cost or quality.

HOW TO PRACTICE GOOD NUTRITION

Not only do supermarkets entice unwary customers to buy high-profit, non-nutritive food loaded with chemicals whose safety is undetermined, but thousands of recipes advise readers to extract and discard nutrients or to destroy them either by long cooking times or by using temperatures that are too high.[31,32] The following sections contain a few ideas on nutrition-wise shopping and cooking.

Nutrition-wise shopping. Look for whole foods free of chemical additives, preservatives, colorants, and artificial flavorings. To protect yourself from unwanted additives, get in the habit of reading labels. Read everything, including the fine print. Labels on foods follow a standard format. Although complete disclosure of the contents is not required by law, labels will at least contain those ingredients which must be listed. Ingredients are listed in decreasing order of predominance. For example, if wheat flour is listed first, it is present in the greatest quantity. Any ingredients listed after wheat flour are present in smaller amounts, decreasing in the order listed on the label.

Get in the habit of looking for hidden sugar. A surprising number of foods contain sugar, including canned soups, sauces, canned vegetables, baked beans, pickles, processed meats, peanut butter, ketchup and other sauces, crackers, mayonnaise, and almost all convenience foods. You may not be able to eliminate all sugar from your diet, but you should be able to reduce your sugar consumption drastically by avoiding those foods known to contain sugar. Sugar masquerades under many disguises to confuse the unwary consumer. Sugar may be listed several times on one label as sucrose, corn syrup, fructose, corn sweeteners, or dextrose. Raw sugar and turbinado sugar are equivalent to brown sugar, both being made from refined white sugar with some molasses added back to give the brown color and distinctive flavor. Incidentally, if you need to use sugar, brown sugar is preferred to white sugar because brown sugar contains trace amounts of chromium, a nutrient now considered essential for metabolizing sugar.

Fresh vegetables are preferred to frozen, and frozen preferred to canned. For salads, you will want to purchase leafy green varieties, such as romaine, green leaf, red tip and bibb. Pale varieties, such as iceberg lettuce, are deficient in nutrients compared to the darker varieties. Purchase cold pressed vegetable oils and prepare your own salad dressings.

Avoid dried fruits and fresh fruits with high sugar content, such as grapes and watermelon. Select instead citrus fruit, apples, bananas, pears and seasonal varieties such as melons and berries.

Labels such as rye flour, wheat flour and white flour are equivalent and of little nutritive value. Look for breads made with wholewheat flour or other whole grains. Consider buying wholegrain flours and meals to bake your own bread.

Avoid the overprocessed, oversweetened, overpriced dry breakfast cereals and also the quick-cooking variety. Try new grains such as unbolted cornmeal, bulgur, millet, triticale and brown rice. Unrefined grains cook almost as quickly as their refined counterparts and are better sources of protein, vitamins and minerals. Look for ingredients to make your own homemade granola.

The biggest supermarket bargain in foods are the legumes: peas, beans and lentils. They can be used in many creative ways for delicious and nutritious meals.

Look for wheat germ, nutritional yeast and non-instant powdered milk. These foods can be added to a variety of dishes such as breads, cereals, soups, stews and meat loaf to enhance nutritional quality. Yogurt is another valuable food, well tolerated by many persons who cannot digest milk.

Nutrition-wise cooking. Food preparation techniques should be adopted that preserve as many nutrients as possible. For example, since heat and light destroy many nutrients rapidly, glass lids and glass cooking pots which expose food to light at high temperatures are not recommended. Essential amino acids begin to break apart when proteins are cooked too long or at too high temperatures, reducing protein quality. Therefore, meat, poultry and fish should be cooked for as short a time at as low a temperature as possible.[32]

Salt should not be used in cooking unless the nutrients are to be drawn into the cooking liquid, as in the preparation of soups, where the liquid is eaten. If no salt is used in cooking vegetables, the flavor remains in the vegetable and little or no salt need be added at the table.[32]

Steaming or stir frying quickly in hot oil are recommended techniques for cooking many vegetables. Exposing the cut edges of vegetables to heat destroys nutrients. On the other hand, the longer cooking time required for larger pieces also destroys nutrients. Compromise so that vegetables cook reasonably quickly. Properly cooked vegetables retain firm texture, bright color and excellent flavor.[32]

Any liquid left from cooking should be saved. This liquid contains many valuable nutrients and can be used in a number of ways: for example, to make delicious soups, or as the liquid for cooking rice or pasta, or in making bread.[32]

Learn to use nutritional additives such as nutritional yeast, wheat germ, and powdered milk in recipes to provide extra nutritive value to make meals. Yogurt is an excellent food and easy to make at home with store-bought, unpasteurized, unsweetened yogurt for a starter. Alfalfa seeds, mung beans, and other dried beans and seeds can be readily sprouted at home. Sprouts are a concentrated source of nutrients and delicious in salads, sandwiches, or served with cooked vegetables.

When care is exercised in cooking so that as many of the nutrients are preserved as possible, when whole grains, fresh fruits and vegetables are used, when complementarity is exercised in making the entire meal as nutritious as possible, food is so complete and so satisfying that smaller portions of food are needed. The end result is better nutrition at less cost. Good health is a real bargain.

NUTRITIONAL SUPPLEMENTS

Alcoholics generally exhibit multiple nutritional deficiencies and may need dietary regimens containing far in excess of *R*ecommended *D*aily *A*llowances.[16] Because of losses in nutrients due to shipping, processing, and subsequent losses from cooking in spite of prudent food preparation, even a careful selection of wholesome, unprocessed food may not provide adequate nutrition.[14] Additional nutrients in the form of vitamin and mineral supplements may also be desirable. Research has shown that with adequate nutrition (that is, a good diet and vitamin and mineral supplements) sobriety can be maintained. A formulation similar to that used successfully in one study is shown in Table 1.[21] Because of highly distinctive individual requirements and differences in absorption of nutrients from food, the amounts shown in Table 1 should be considered as a general guideline only.

All minerals and some vitamins accumulate in the body if taken in excess of the amount which can be utilized. For this reason, it is preferable to purchase several different supplements rather than choosing a supplement formulated to contain all nutrients in one large capsule or tablet. The following supplements are suggested: vitamin C tablets, vitamin E capsules, vitamin A and D capsules, B complex tablets, stress tablets (a high potency B complex supplement sometimes containing vitamin C), and multimineral tablets.

Vitamin E is not toxic, and the amount taken could gradually be increased to 800 IU daily. If unsaturated fats are added to the diet, sufficient vitamin E should be taken. However, if any heart problems exist, vitamin E should be started in very small quantities, perhaps 30 IU per day, and only very gradually increased. If pain results, the dosage should be reduced and your physician consulted. Although natural and synthetic vitamins are considered equivalent in most cases, only natural vitamin E is completely biologically active.

Amino acid chelated minerals are the most readily assim-

TABLE 1.

An Example of A Nutritional Supplement Program

VITAMINS

	B-Complex (6 Tablets Per Day)	*Stress Tablets (6 Tablets Per Day)*	*Total Amount Per Day*
B1	5 mg	30 mg	35 mg
B2	5 mg	30 mg	35 mg
B6	5 mg	30 mg	35 mg
Niacinamide	50 mg	300 mg	350 mg
B12	15 mcg	75 mcg	90 mcg
Biotin	25 mcg	75 mcg	100 mcg
Folic acid	.1 mg	.3 mg	.4 mg
Pantothenic acid	100 mg	300 mg	400 mg
Choline	500 mg	150 mg	650 mg
Inositol	1000 mg	300 mg	1300 mg
Para-amino-benzoic acid (PABA)	30 mg	90 mg	120 mg
Vitamin C		1500 mg	1500 mg

Vitamin E (d-alpha tocopherol)	100 IU
Vitamin A	10,000 IU
Vitamin D	400 IU

MINERALS

Calcium	1,000 mg
Magnesium	500 mg
Iodine	225 mcg
Iron	20 mg
Copper	1 mg
Zinc	22.5 mg
Manganese	10 mg
Potassium	95 mg
Chromium	100 mcg
Selenium	7.5 mcg

ilated form of all mineral supplements. All the minerals shown in Table 1 can be obtained in one multimineral formulation. Research has shown that liver damaged from alcohol abuse stores iron. Since excess iron can be toxic, no more than 20 mg per day, the amount shown in Table 1, should be taken.[16]

The B vitamins, shown in Table 1 as B complex and stress tablets, are water-soluble and do not accumulate in the body. In the body, B vitamins act as coenzymes; that is, they are parts of enzymes. Enzymes are catalysts which speed up chemical reactions. Persons with either inborn enzyme deficiencies or acquired nutritional deficiencies which may cause inability to synthesize certain enzymes, need B vitamins. The amounts shown in Table 1 are reasonable ones with which to start. If renewed energy is not experienced within a few weeks, the amount of B complex or stress tablets can be increased gradually. Stop increasing the dosage when adding more B vitamins no longer seems to produce any change in mood or energy. The amount should then be decreased gradually until a decrease in energy level is noticed. Then increase the dosage to your maximum energy level; this will be the amount of B vitamins you need. Maintain this dosage for about six months. At that time, your B vitamin need could be reassessed by repeating the above procedure.[33]

Because smoking depletes the body of vitamin C, those who persist in smoking should take additional vitamin C in the amount of 1500 mg per day for each pack of cigarettes smoked each day.

If improved health does not result from improved diet and use of vitamin and mineral supplements, faulty absorption may be a problem. The various digestive aids available at health food stores help break down food to increase absorption in the digestive tract.

It is best to take supplements in divided doses, one-third at each meal. However, if you are not able to take your supplements when away from home or if you are likely to forget them, then take them all in the morning.

Some persons are able to begin their vitamin and mineral regimen all at once, while others experience digestive disturbances with this approach. It may be best to introduce supplements slowly, allowing the body to become tolerant. For example, vitamin E could be introduced first, followed by C, then A and D, with B complex next, then stress tablets, and lastly, minerals. Add one new nutrient or group of nutrients each day, perhaps at breakfast. Take one-third of the total amount you are planning to take for the entire day. After you have introduced one-third of all the supplements in the morning, add another one-third, one at a time, to the evening meal. Finally, add the remaining one-third at lunch time, again one at a time. If at any time you feel that any one of the supplements is causing digestive problems, try to decide if the problem has been caused by introducing it too rapidly or if perhaps your body is sensitive to that supplement. Sometimes there may be intolerance to one brand of supplement because of a particular filler used in the formulation, but another brand may be well tolerated.

GUIDELINES FOR RECOVERY

- Eat three meals a day and snacks between meals.
- Avoid caffeine, sugar and other processed foods.
- Take vitamin and mineral supplements according to your individual needs.
- Never let yourself get hungry.
- Learn techniques to control stress.
- Remember to obtain extra nourishment whenever you are under stress.
- Exercise moderately.

RECOMMENDED READING LIST

Davis, A. 1970. *Let's Cook It Right.* New York, NY: New American Library.

Goldbeck, N. and Goldbeck, D. 1976. *The Supermarket Handbook.* New York, NY: New American Library.

Hoffer, A. and Walker, W. 1978. *Orthomolecular Nutrition.* New Canaan, CT: Keats Publishing.

Hunter, Beatrice Trum. 1969. *The Natural Foods Cookbook.* New York, NY: Fireside Press (Simon & Schuster).

Lappe, F. 1975. *Diet for a Small Planet.* New York, NY: Ballantine Books.

Passwater, R. 1977. *Super-Nutrition.* New York, NY: Pocket Books.

Williams, R.J. 1977. *The Wonderful World Within You.* New York, NY: Bantam Books.

REFERENCES

1. Keller, M., and Rosenberg, S.S. (eds.). 1973. *Alcohol and Health: Report From the Secretary of Health, Education, and Welfare.* New York, NY: Charles Scribner's Sons.
2. Hamilton, M.H. *Austin-American Statesman.* May 26, 1980, p. D1.
3. Grabbs, J. 1980. *The Magazine of the Texas Commission of Alcoholism* 6: 22-23.
4. Lieber, C.S. 1976. *Scientific American* 234:25-33.
5. Witti, F.P. 1978. *FDA Consumer.* HEW Publication No. (FDA) 78-1047.
6. Emrick, C.D. 1975. *Journal of Studies on Alcohol* 36:52-61.
7. Mosher, V. *et al.* 1975. *Journal of Studies on Alcohol* 36:1277-1281.
8. Philpott, W.H. *Texas Key Newsletter,* February 1975.
9. Murphree, H.B. 1971. In *Biological Basis of Alcoholism,* Y. Israel and J. Mardones (eds.). New York, NY: Wiley-Interscience.
10. Davis, A. 1965. *Let's Get Well: A Practical Guide to Renewed Health Through Nutrition.* New York, NY: Harcourt, Brace, and World.
11. Gilbert, R.M. 1976. *Journal of Studies on Alcohol* 37:284-297.
12. Register, U.D. *et al.* 1972. *The Journal of the American Dietetic Association* 61:159-162.
13. Williams, R.J. 1947. *Quarterly Journal of Studies on Alcohol* 4:567-587.
14. Williams, R.J. 1977. *The Wonderful World Within You.* New York, NY: Bantam Books.
15. Williams, R.J. 1967. *You Are Extraordinary.* New York, NY: Pyramid Books.
16. Roe, D. 1979. *Alcohol and the Diet.* Westport, CT: The Avi Publishing Company.
17. Williams, R.J. Paper presented at the National Academy of Science, October 1971.
18. Lester, D. and Greenberg, L.A. 1952. *Quarterly Journal of Studies on Alcohol* 13:553-560.
19. Rogers, L.L. *et al.* 1955. *Journal of Biological Chemistry* 503:214.
20. Roe, D. 1976. *Drug-Induced Nutritional Deficiencies.* Westport, CT: The Avi Publishing Co.
21. Guenther, R. 1980. *The Effect of Nutritional Therapy on Rehabilitation of Alcoholics.* Ann Arbor, MI: University Microfilms International.
22. Hawkins, D. and Pauling, L. 1973. *Orthomolecular Psychiatry.* San Francisco, CA: W.H. Freeman and Company.

23. Lear, L. 1976. *Prevention* 28:157-166.
24. Harris, R.S. and Karmer, E. 1975. *Nutritional Evaluation of Food Processing,* 2nd ed. Westport, CT: The Avi Publishing Co.
25. Lappe, F.M. 1975. *Diet for a Small Planet.* New York, NY: Ballantine Books.
26. Passwater, R. 1981. *Evening Primrose Oil: Its Amazing Nutrients and the Health Benefits They Can Give You.* New Canaan, CT: Keats Publishing.
27. Schroeder, H. 1971. *The American Journal of Clinical Nutrition* 24:562-573.
28. Pfeiffer, C.C. 1978. *Zinc and Other Micro-Nutrients.* New Canaan, CT: Keats Publishing.
29. Church, C.F. and Church, H.N. *Food Values of Portions Commonly Used,* 12th ed. New York, NY: J.B. Lippincott Co.
30. Shannon, I.L. 1977. *Brand Name Guide to Sugar.* Chicago, IL: Nelson-Hall.
31. Goldbeck, N. and Goldbeck, D. 1976. *The Supermarket Handbook.* New York, NY: New American Library.
32. Davis, A. 1970. *Let's Cook It Right.* New York, NY: New American Library.
33. Passwater, R. 1977. *Super-Nutrition.* New York, NY: Pocket Books.